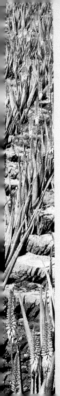

Understanding
Aloe Vera

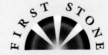

Contents

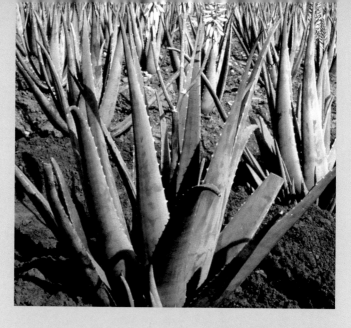

1

Introducing Aloe Vera

Aloe vera, the true aloe, is properly called Aloe Barbadensis Miller. Medicinally, it is the most powerful of all the aloe varieties – of which there are some 350 in the world.

Although the aloe plant looks like a cactus, it is actually a succulent and, being a member of the lily family, it is related to onions, garlic and asparagus.

All aloes originated in Africa, but they have spread across the world wherever they have found the right climate and conditions – sunny, dry places where there is never a hint of frost (aloe's worst enemy).

NATURAL PROTECTION
Aloe vera is a very successful plant, well protected against its enemies – rodents, insects and birds. Just below the rind of the plant is a very bitter, noxious sap that deters any animal that tries to eat it.

Aloe plants can reproduce both sexually and asexually, depending upon the

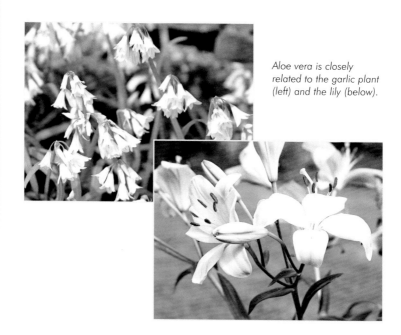

Aloe vera is closely related to the garlic plant (left) and the lily (below).

conditions, and they can survive for several months without water. Aloe has the ability to shut itself down and close its stomata – little holes in the leaves – through which it normally loses water vapour.

HEALING PLANT

Aloe has achieved some remarkable nicknames from around the world. These include:

- Medicine plant
- Miracle plant
- Silent healer
- Wand of heaven
- Burn plant.

The name 'burn plant' owes its origin to aloe's remarkable ability to relieve burn pain; anyone who has had freshly expelled gel from the leaf smeared over their sunburnt skin will testify to this. Indeed, aloe contains remarkable pain-relieving properties, which work almost instantaneously. Further applications of the leaf gel also help to speed up the healing of the damaged skin.

7

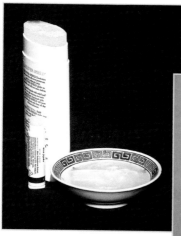

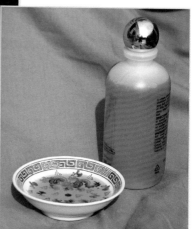

The cosmetics industry has been quick to see the potential of aloe vera.

COMMERCIAL PRODUCTS

There are many uses for topically applied aloe – a fact well known to the cosmetic industry. A number of products today use the tag 'with aloe vera', ranging from make-up and bathing products, through to washing powder and detergents. As well as being applied topically, the gel or juice of aloe vera can also be drunk as a tonic.

With so many applications for this most versatile plant, it should come as no surprise that aloe vera has remained popular throughout history.

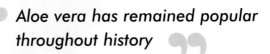

Aloe vera has remained popular throughout history

2 A Brief History

The name 'aloe vera' is probably derived from the Arabic 'alloeh' or the Syrian 'alwai', which mean 'a shining bitter substance'. These names refer to the laxative properties of bitter aloes.

ANCIENT HISTORY
A famous papyrus discovered in Thebes in 1858, which dates to the reign of the Pharaoh Amen-Hotep in 1552 BC, lists the use of aloe both in drugs and cosmetics, demonstrating the use of aloe vera over the preceding 2,000 years.

Over the centuries, aloe vera has been known to many different cultures, from the Ancient Greeks and Romans, to Babylonian, Indian and Chinese peoples. It was also well known to the ancient physicians, such as Hippocrates in AD 70-90 and the Greek physician Dioscorides, who wrote one of the greatest medical books ever written – *De Materia Medica*.

FABLES AND MYTHS

There are many myths surrounding aloe vera's history, such as those concerning Egyptian queens Cleopatra and Nefertiti, who were thought to have used aloes as part of their beauty regimes.

In 333 BC Alexander the Great was reported to have fought a battle to capture the island of Socotra in the Indian Ocean. He needed the aloe supplies to treat his wounded soldiers. The truth of these legends will never be known.

ALOE IN BRITAIN

Dioscorides' *De Materia Medica* was translated into English in 1655. Traders first brought aloe to London in 1693.

By 1850 aloe vera was in widespread use. The sap of the plant, aloin (commonly called 'bitter aloes'), was sold as a tonic to assist digestion, or in larger doses as a strong laxative.

Today, aloe products remain as popular as ever, illustrating that this natural product has been valued by makind for more than two millennia.

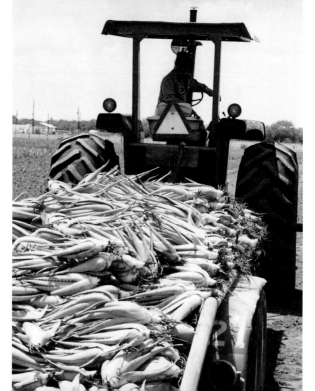

The healing power of herbs is well documented in folklore. Aloe has been used for more than two millennia, and today it is harvested around the world.

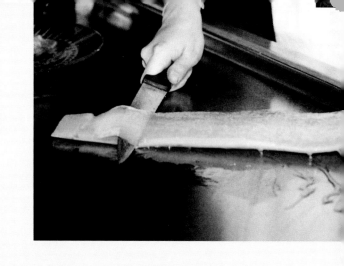

Composition And Chemistry

The aloe vera plant takes four to five years to reach maturity. When fully matured, its leaves – which grow from a short stem – are about 60cm in length and about 8-10cm wide at the base.

Aloe vera is a perennial, living for about 12 years, but the leaves can be harvested from about two years of age.

FLOWERS

The flower stem develops from the middle of the mass of dark-green leaves. It reaches about 90cm in length and produces long, tubular yellow flowers.

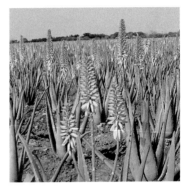

Aloe vera produces long, tubular-shaped yellow flowers.

The flowers are often pollinated by humming birds, but the plant can also produce little suckers or 'pups' that grow from the base of the mother plant and are genetically identical. These spread as a clump, or they become detached and are spread by the wind.

LEAVES

The leaves taper to a point and possess soft, marginal spines. If the stem is cut across, the leaves can be seen growing in a rosette pattern.

The leaf comprises four main constituents: the rind, the sap, the mucilage and the inner gel.

The rind of the aloe vera leaf is dark green and waxy. Below it are vascular bundles or tubules containing the sap or 'aloin'.

Inside this is a mucilage layer, rich in polysaccharide sugars, which surrounds the inner gel or parenchyma (the water-storage organ of the plant).

ALOE PROPERTIES

There are more than 75 known ingredients in the aloe vera leaf, but not all of them have been identified. There are probably others still to be discovered. The solid fraction of the plant only forms 0.5-1.5 per cent (98.5-99.5 per cent being water) and the constituents can be broken down into several main groups:

❶ **Lignin:** A totally inert, cellulose-based substance when swallowed, it is believed to give topical products their ability to penetrate deep into the skin.

❷ **Saponins:** These are soapy substances that are capable of cleansing. They posses natural antiseptic properties.

❸ **Anthraquinones:** These are found only in the sap. They are what gives bitter aloes its laxative effect. It is interesting to know that these substances are also found in senna and cascara, which are commonly used as laxatives, and even in rhubarb.

④Minerals: Sodium, potassium, magnesium, calcium, zinc, copper, iron and chromium. The only important mineral absent is selenium, which is a very important antioxidant mineral. Ideally, therefore, a selenium supplement should be added when taking an aloe vera product.

⑤Vitamins: These comprise mainly the antioxidant vitamins A, C and E, together with the B group, even having a trace of vitamin B12, which is very rarely found in plants. The only important vitamin that aloe vera does not have is vitamin D. Consequently, exposure to sufficient sunshine is important, as this will provide enough vitamin D from the skin.

⑥Amino acids: The human body requires 20 amino acids and aloe vera possesses 19 of them. It also provides seven of the so-called 'essential' amino acids that have to be taken in as food because the body cannot manufacture them.

❼Enzymes: Aloe vera contains two main types of enzyme – anti-inflammatory enzymes and digestive enzymes. People who drink aloe vera regularly tend to absorb food better, particularly protein. I also believe that aloe vera helps people to absorb drugs more efficiently – something that they need to be aware of, as they may need less conventional medication when on aloe vera.

❽Sugars: Aloe vera contains both monosaccharides, such as glucose, and polysaccharides. Of the latter, the most significant is the long chain sugar composed of glucose and mannose molecules, which is capable of affecting the immune system. This is called glucomannose, polymannose, or, colloquially, acemannan.

❾Plant sterols: Aloe vera contains three plant sterols,

all of which provide anti-inflammatory effects.

⑩ Salicylic acid: This is metabolised in the body. It is aspirin-like in its action and produces pain-killing and anti-inflammatory effects.

PERFECT BALANCE

You might be surprised at how such a small amount of aloe vera can produce such a pronounced effect. The reason for this is that all the substances contained in aloe vera work together in perfect balance and harmony.

This is known as a 'synergistic' action, which basically means that the effect of the whole group is much greater than the sum of the effects of each separate group. While this concept cannot be proven, most herbalists accept it as the only explanation.

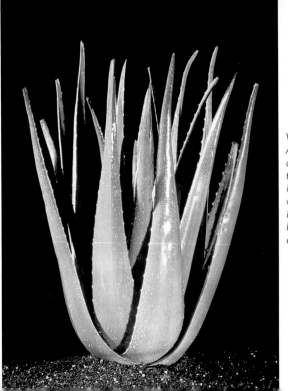

Wonder plant: Aloe vera contains more than 75 ingredients, all of which are important for human health and well-being.

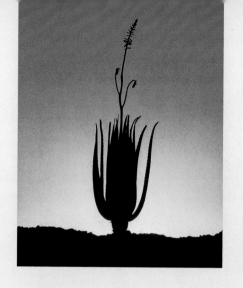

4

How Aloe Vera Works

Aloe vera works in two main areas: firstly on body surfaces and membranes (referred to anatomically as epithelial tissue) and secondly on the immune system.

It is remarkably effective in both these areas, but it is important to realise that aloe vera is not a panacea or 'cure all'.

EFFECTS ON TISSUE

An epithelium is defined as 'a layer of cells lining the surface of the body or a cavity that connects with it'. The skin is our largest epithelial surface, and both the hairs and nails that grow from it are epithelial in origin and so are affected by aloe vera.

Epithelium becomes a mucous membrane inside the mouth, nose, sinuses, and throat. Epithelium also lines the gullet, the stomach, the intestines, the genital tract and the lungs. Where any of these tissues are damaged, aloe vera can exert a remarkable effect,

23

helping to regenerate tissue and promote healing.

People who drink aloe vera regularly often find their hair grows faster and that they need to visit the hairdresser more often. Hair also becomes stronger and more luxuriant. In the quest for solutions to split ends and fewer broken nails, aloe vera can play a valuable role.

It possesses a powerful anti-inflammatory effect and broad anti-microbial activity. When applied topically, it has the ability to penetrate deeply into the skin, where it stimulates the fibroblasts that produce collagen and elastin. It encourages them to replicate themselves faster than they would normally. This speeds up the healing of damaged skin or membranes. Research has shown that aloe vera can increase the rate of healing by about a third.

It is no surprise then that hair and beauty products containing aloe vera are so popular.

THE ANTI-AGEING COSMETIC PROPERTIES OF ALOE VERA

- Gives a smoother look to the skin by improving cohesion where superficial skin cells are stuck together.
- Improves skin texture with its intense moisturisation.
- Reduces the effects of ultraviolet light by strengthening the skin's immune response.
- Reduces the tendency to form 'liver spots' or 'age spots'. In some cases, it can even cause existing ones to disappear.
- Reduces wrinkle formation by improving the replication of skin fibroblasts (the cells that make collagen and elastin fibres).

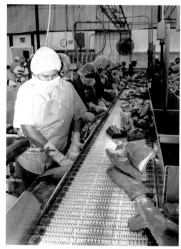

Aloe vera is widely used in the cosmetics industry, being processed to produce a multitude of products.

EFFECTS ON THE IMMUNE SYSTEM

Aloe vera works on the immune system because of the long chain sugar acemannan, which is found in the mucilage layer of the leaf.

Acemannan can be absorbed whole through specialised cells lining the small bowel. Once absorbed, it can affect the chemical messenger, or cytokine system, which regulates the immune response. Laboratory research has shown that, in some cases, acemannan enhances the immune response, while in other cases, it can be seen to slow it down. Hence this sugar is known as an immuno-modulator. Not many substances can qualify for this description.

FOOD FOR THOUGHT

Apart from affecting the body's tissues and immune system, aloe vera can be taken as a source of food. It provides a range of micronutrients when drunk, as well as trace elements that are now rapidly becoming deficient from our diet.

The areas where aloe grows – often in dried-up sea beds and river beds – are places rich in minerals. The aloe plant is able to absorb these minerals from the ground and make them available to us when we drink the juice of the plant. This improves the efficiency of all our enzyme systems, which rely on these trace elements. As a result, our whole body is able to function more efficiently.

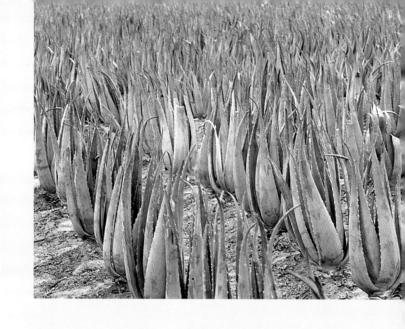

Common Problems

There are a number of common complaints that aloe vera can play a valuable part in helping to manage.

SKIN CONDITIONS

Aloe vera has the capacity to heal damaged skin. By drinking the juice of the plant, all the micronutrients and trace elements needed to produce new skin cells can be ingested naturally.

By applying aloe vera topically, the healing process is stimulated by reducing inflammation, preventing infection, and encouraging the growth of skin cells called fibroblasts. These fibres are laid down in wounds and damaged skin. They facilitate healing by contracting, closing the wound. They also act as a framework for new skin cells to grow over.

The effects of aloe vera on skin has long made it popular with the cosmetics industry (see page 25), which promotes it as a means of helping people to stay young and beautiful. However, aloe vera's remarkable healing properties mean that it can be a significant help in managing common skin complaints. These include:

- **Eczema and dermatitis:** Both these conditions respond well to aloe vera, especially the chronic variety where there is often an allergic element. From my own experience, I have also found that juvenile or atopic eczemas respond particularly well to aloe vera combined with moisturisers (although the sugars in aloe vera gel act as moisturisers in their own right). Children with this type of eczema tend to scratch a lot, even in their sleep. Since aloe vera contains a natural anti-histamine, itchiness can be reduced, giving the rash a better chance to settle down. This is important, because when eczema is scratched by dirty finger nails, there is considerable risk of infection, which will cause the eczema to spread very rapidly.

- **Psoriasis:** This is actually a disorder of the immune system. Psoriasis is a general medical condition that can manifest itself as a skin complaint. There is plenty of anecdotal evidence to support the fact that some types of psoriasis respond excellently to drinking aloe vera and applying it topically. In a few cases, it completely disappears, although this is not true for all cases.

A clinical trial carried out in Sweden has demonstrated the effectiveness of a topical aloe product on psoriasis. It showed an 83 per cent cure rate for those using aloe vera extract cream compared to 6.6 per cent of those using a placebo.

- **Acne:** Common acne (*Vulgaris*) and rosacea (found in older people) respond to topical applications of aloe vera. It can reduce inflammation, making the skin appear less red, especially in rosacea. It also

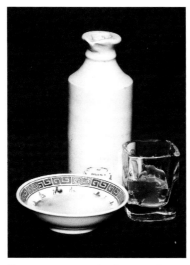

Aloe vera creams and gels can work wonders on skin conditions, such as acne.

has the ability to kill the bacteria that are part of the cause of common acne. In addition, aloe can also reduce the tendency towards scarring, which is very important for acne sufferers.

- **Fungal infections:** Complaints such as ringworm and athlete's foot respond very well to topically applied aloe. This is because aloe contains properties that can kill fungi and yeasts.

- **Chronic ulcers and bed sores:** These are notoriously difficult to treat, often because there is an underlying problem with the blood supply to the affected area. However, where the blood supply is just about adequate, an occlusive dressing with an appropriate aloe product can often stimulate healing. Such treatment needs to be carried out persistently, though, in order to achieve healing.

DISORDERS OF THE IMMUNE SYSTEM

Aloe has a powerful anti-inflammatory action when ingested. As a result, it can have a significant effect on conditions related to the immune system.

- **Rheumatoid arthritis:** In many cases, the sufferer is able to reduce their dependence on conventional medication, and, consequently, are subjected to less risk from side effects.
- **Lupus:** This connective tissue

disorder can benefit from taking aloe in some cases.

- **Ulcerative colitis and Crohn's disease:** These are inflammatory bowel conditions and both may benefit from taking aloe vera. A recent British clinical trial has just demonstrated the superiority of an aloe vera drink over a placebo in the management of ulcerative colitis.
- **Irritable bowel syndrome:** Conventional medicine accepts that there is no single successful treatment for this complex condition. However, I have found that more than half the patients I have treated have benefited considerably from taking aloe vera (although this is not to say that it can help all cases).

The symptoms of IBS include griping pains and a change in bowel habit (usually diarrhoea), varying from mild, infrequent attacks to severe and socially handicapping ones.

IBS is a functional condition – there is nothing pathologically wrong with the bowel when looked at on operation or at post mortem; it just does not work properly. I believe aloe vera helps because it regulates movement in the bowel, making it contract and relax in a rhythmical fashion. This would have the natural consequence of reducing the tendency to colicky pain.

Furthermore, aloe vera regulates gut flora. An overgrowth of yeast may be a factor in IBS, and, if the yeast is controlled, symptoms should reduce.

I believe that the immune-balancing properties of aloe help to make people feel better 'in themselves', which has a knock-on effect on their emotional well-being. As stress is believed to be a factor that can trigger IBS, an improved feeling of well-being should help to minimise attacks.

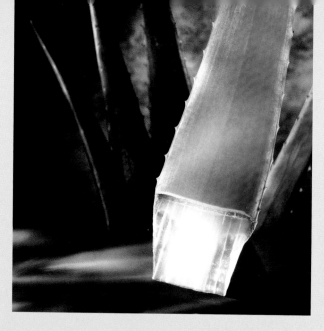

6 Using Aloe Vera

There are many different types of aloe vera products available. These range from tablets and capsules to drinks, lotions and cosmetics.

There are refined drinks marketed as juices, and less refined ones marketed as gels.

Of the topical products, there are creams, lotions, sprays and cosmetics, as well as shampoos, deodorants and gargles.

Occasionally, aloe vera is impregnated in tissues, and it has even been put in babies' nappies, ladies' tights and latex examination gloves.

The latest significant addition to the range of products containing aloe vera is washing powder. Indeed, aloe vera seems to have become a bit of a sales buzzword.

A NOTE OF CAUTION

Unfortunately, many of the products claiming to include aloe vera contain so little as to make them ineffectual. When looking for aloe products always try to find one where the main ingredient of the product is aloe vera, with other

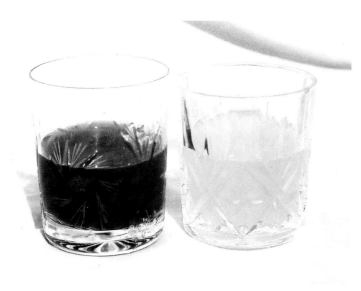

Drinks containing aloe vera are made in different flavours.

additives also included – not the other way around. Look for the International Aloe Science Council seal of approval on the product, and disregard cheap tablets of dried aloe vera, which are pretty useless.

FINDING THE RIGHT PRODUCT

To be effective, a product must contain a significant amount of aloe vera that has been manufactured and stabilised in such a way that it has not undergone excessive heating, filtration or concentration.

When using a herbal extract, try to find one that is as near as possible to the natural plant. My own preference would be to find products containing a cold, stabilised gel, unfiltered and unconcentrated.

DANGERS OF FILTRATION

We do not know every single constituent of aloe vera. Therefore, it is possible that vital ingredients could be lost through the filtration process.

Many products claiming to

contain aloe vera are produced using filtration, which is largely done to extract the contaminant aloin. Unfortunately, this process could mean that other, unknown but important, substances could well be filtered out at the same time.

Products that are produced by the whole leaf method – where the whole plant is cut off at the base and then macerated – have to be passed through a series of increasingly fine filters, eventually being filtered through carbon. This produces a very watery product with absolutely no aloin in it.

Other products are produced by a different method, known as the filleting process. Individual leaves of the plant are cut off and put through machines that are set to squeeze out the gel, leaving the sap and rind behind. These products contain a very small amount of aloin, but the amount is insignificant. Indeed, it has been suggested that a small amount of aloin is

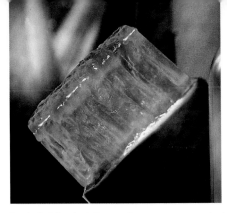

Be wary of the tag 'with aloe vera'. It is better to buy a product that is mainly aloe vera, such as this aloe cube, rather than a product that merely claims to contain some aloe vera.

beneficial – helping to improve absorption from the gut. One could say, for example, that a small dose of aspirin is beneficial, especially if you are suffering from a headache, whereas a large dose would obviously kill you.

SUMMARY

It is down to the individual to decide what product to choose, but it is wise to be cautious of the 'with aloe vera' tag.

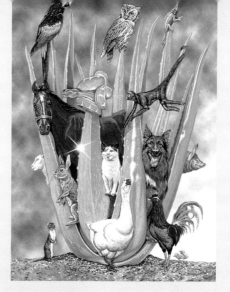

7

Animals
And Aloe Vera

With vets' bills escalating, it is hardly surprising that farmers, pet owners and those involved with horses are anxious to try treating the animals in their care with effective natural products whenever possible.

Many people who take care of animals do not wish to use powerful drugs unnecessarily because of the various, and sometimes unpleasant, side effects they can cause. Nor do they wish to subject their much-loved pets to chemicals unless it is unaviodable. This is where aloe vera can be of huge benefit.

A NATURAL ALTERNATIVE
If you are interested in using aloe vera to treat your animals, please check the Further Reading section in this book (page 60). David Urch's definitive work on the subject of veterinary applications for aloe vera is a 'must read'.

ITCHING

Aloe vera has proven healing properties, and, taken orally, aloe is a natural anti-pruritic. It contains a naturally occurring histamine inhibitor, so it can reduce the itching associated with many skin complaints, especially allergic dermatitis.

Trying to prevent animals from scratching and exacerbating an existing condition can be extremely difficult – most dog owners are familiar with the cumbersome Elizabethan collar. A natural product that can alleviate itching can only be good news.

TOPICAL PRODUCTS

Aloe vera spray, soap, gel and propolis cream can be used to treat various inflammatory skin conditions, such as dermatitis, eczema, abscesses, boils and infected insect bites. Fungal infections, such as ringworm, can also be helped, together with traumatic abrasions and ulceration from a badly fitting harness, for example.

Various kinds of wounds, as

well as ulcers and burns, will also heal much more quickly when dressed with aloe vera.

It is generally found that, with the aloe vera healing process, there is minimal scar formation, and, when new fur or hair appears, the re-growth will be the original colour rather than white, which is often the case. This is a major plus where show animals are concerned.

FOOD PRODUCTS
The elements necessary to

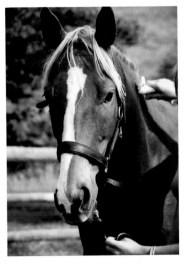

A topical application of aloe gel can be used on an infected insect bite.

produce healthy skin cells are supplied to an area via the bloodstream. Adding aloe vera gel to animal feed can help this process. However, it can be problematic when it comes to cats, as they are notoriously fussy and may not like the taste. One solution is to paint it on their fur, which they will soon lick clean.

FIGHTING FATIGUE

Animals, like humans, are prone to viral infections, especially the influenza-like viruses. While most animals make a full recovery, a small percentage go on to develop a form of post-viral fatigue syndrome, similar to ME (myalgic encephalitis), which affects humans. Such animals become lethargic and tire easily when exercising.

With horses this condition can be particularly pronounced and debilitating. Conventional treatment has shown a marked lack of success, with the result that many horses are unable to return to their previous activities, such as racing, dressage or eventing.

Unlike humans, horses affected by this condition develop changes in the blood. Their white blood-cell count drops, sometimes to almost fatal levels.

Equine vet Peter Green once had 14 of his animals develop post-viral lethargy, following an attack of influenza. Using aloe vera gel, he managed to return 11 of his 14 horses back to full health – something previously unheard of. The blood tests showed that, prior to treatment, all the affected horses showed a reduced white cell count, but following treatment, the 11 animals that had recovered showed a return to normal levels.

It is most likely that Green achieved such remarkable effects using aloe vera because of the immuno-modulating effect of the long chain sugar acemannan, which is derived from the mucilage layer of the aloe vera plant and found in the gel that Green used.

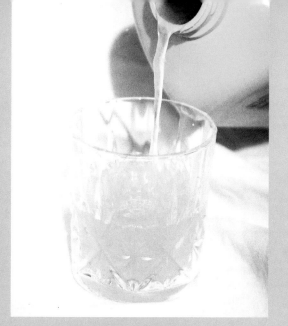

8

Case Studies

The following case studies illustrate ways in which aloe vera can be used to help common complaints.

❶ ARTHRITIS

Jenny had suffered from severe arthritis for more than 20 years. She was finding it hard to manage the pain of her condition, and it was waking her several times during the night. She was also having to give up many of her daily activities and hobbies as a result.

After being recommended aloe vera gel for her condition, Jenny decided to give it a go. Within a matter of days, she noticed a significant reduction in her level of pain.

Now, two years on, Jenny is managing to live a virtually pain-free life during the day, and she has found it far easier to get unbroken sleep through the night as well.

❷ BURNS

Toddler Bethany received extensive burns to her body when she accidentally got too close to a fire.

After weeks of intense hospital treatment, Bethany's burns were eventually covered with bandages and the healing process was allowed to begin.

Bethany's parents had been told not to remove the bandages or to apply anything to Bethany's skin. However, they were anxious to keep their daughter as pain-free as possible, and preferred, where possible, to use natural alternatives to powerful medication. After careful consultation with Bethany's doctors, it was agreed that Bethany could take aloe vera gel – well known for its healing properties – in oral form only.

After six weeks, Bethany's bandages were ready to be removed. Bethany's parents were warned that this could prove extremely painful, and that Bethany may need to be heavily sedated. However, the bandages came off relatively easily, and both parents and hospital staff were amazed at what they saw – nearly all of Bethany's burns had healed over with dry scar tissue. There were no weeping sores or blisters to be seen.

Today, Bethany's entire family drink aloe vera gel on a daily basis. They believe it is the reason that everyone in their family is hardly ever ill, and they remain deeply grateful for the healing help it gave their little daughter.

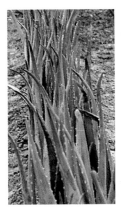

Healing help: Bethany's family believe that gel taken from the aloe vera plant helped their daughter to recover from extensive burns.

❸ COLD SORES

Like many people, Louise had suffered from cold sores throughout most of her life. While it is not considered a serious medical condition, it was beginning to affect her confidence – particularly as they always seemed to flare up at important times or when Louise was on her favourite ski-ing holidays.

Various conventional remedies failed to achieve results, and, although she was not entirely convinced about the merits of aloe vera, Louise decided to treat her cold sores with aloe vera out of desperation.

Louise began using aloe vera soap and applying sunscreen and lip salve made from aloe vera. After eight days on one of her ski-ing holidays, Louise became a convert. She says, "I now need no more proof – each day I wake up with beautiful lips."

4 ECZEMA

Eight-year-old Julie had a common form of childhood eczema, which she had suffered from since she was a toddler. The condition had become steadily worse over a period of years, interrupting Julie's sleep and driving her mad with intense itching.

Julie's parents tried numerous remedies, from traditional medication, including steroid cream, to alternative therapies, such as homoeopathy. Nothing worked. Then Julie's mother discovered a type of aloe vera cream.

She says, "I noticed a difference almost immediately. The rash lost its 'raggedy' appearance and the itching stopped straight away. After four days, the eczema went completely. Now, if I see any tell-tale signs, I just dab on some cream and it nips it in the bud."

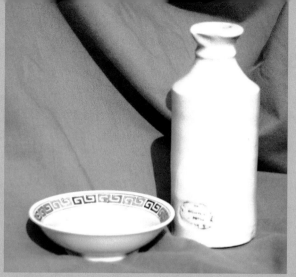

9

The Future
Of Aloe Vera

The properties of aloe vera have been known to ancient cultures for thousands of years.

However, apart from the old 'bitter aloes', it has really only been used in the West over the last 10-15 years.

During this time its popularity has increased enormously, exemplified by the number of products that now contain it. This is partly due to the fact that there has been a sea-change in people's attitudes towards their health and well-being. Many have become frightened of modern medicines and their powerful side effects, and would prefer something that is safer and more natural.

COMPLEMENTARY THERAPY

Interest in complementary therapies, including herbal remedies, has increased enormously, largely due to this shift in attitudes, and I believe that it will continue to do so. Many doctors practising conventional medicine are now beginning to offer complementary alternatives.

Herbs such as St. John's Wort are now being used for depression, Saw Palmetto can be taken for prostate problems, and Fever Few is an effective treatment for migraine. All these natural remedies have been shown to be effective, and they have the added advantage of being cheaper and safer.

In recent years, there has been an increase in the number of clinical trials researching the effectiveness of aloe vera, and, as a result, the medical profession is beginning to recognise this plant's healing properties.

ALOE IN HOSPITALS

Today, aloe vera is being used regularly in the burns units, radiotherapy units, laser clinics and dermatology units of NHS hospitals.

While this trend is new, further trials may see the use of aloe vera extended to other treatments, such as the treatment of chronic venous leg ulcers, or as a soothing agent to reduce immediate post-treatment inflammation and pain (e.g. after laser surgery to a birth mark). The alternative is steroid creams, which are very powerful and efficacious, but, if used regularly over a prolonged period of time, can themselves cause skin damage.

There are now latex surgical gloves lined with freeze-dried aloe vera that becomes hydrated by the sweat produced when the gloves are worn. This causes the skin to be bathed in a soothing aloe vera solution. A considerable number of people are allergic to latex; many, who already have damaged skin, are required to wear latex gloves. In both cases, aloe vera can help to prevent a problem or to treat it.

Disposable latex gloves are used in their millions, and they are still considered to be the best material, although there is a lot of research going on into finding a substance that would cause fewer allergic problems. Aloe vera gloves may offer a partial solution.

The future of aloe vera in medicine is very exciting. With an increasing number of people wishing to take greater responsibility for their own health, aloe vera will have an important role to play in the management of many mild-to-moderate conditions. It can be used quite happily alongside most conventional medicines as well.

CONTRAINDICATIONS

While aloe vera is generally safe to use, some conditions require careful consideration. Drinking aloe vera can affect the following drugs/patients:

- **Anti-coagulants:** These include the popular drug Warfarin. Consult your doctor before beginning to take aloe vera.
- **Drugs for high blood pressure:** Aloe vera may lower blood pressure. Effects are not drastic, but less conventional medicine

may be needed. Patients should discuss their condition with their doctor before taking aloe vera.

- **Diabetics:** Some diabetics find that drinking aloe vera reduces their blood-sugar level. While this is a good effect, it means that the amount of insulin needed may fluctuate. Diabetics should monitor their blood sugar levels closely when taking aloe vera, and should never take anything that could affect their treatment without first discussing it with their doctor.

> *Four vegetables are indispensable for the well-being of man: wheat, the grape, the olive and the aloe. The first nourishes you, the second raises the spirit, the third brings you harmony, and the fourth cures you.*
> Christopher Columbus

Further Information

USEFUL CONTACTS
Dr. Atherton can be contacted at:
Whitings,
Gayhurst,
Newport Pagnell,
Bucks, MK16 8LG.
Email:
doctoratherton@hotmail.com

FURTHER READING
Dr. Peter Atherton
*The Essential Aloe Vera: The
Actions And The Evidence*
1997, Mill Enterprises.

David Urch
*Aloe Vera – Nature's Gift: Aloe Vera
In Veterinary Practice*
1999, Author Publishing Ltd.

REFERENCES
Danhof, I.E. & McAnalley, B.H.
*Stabilised aloe vera – effect on
human skin cells*

Drug & Cosmetic Industry 1983,
133. 52,54, pp105-106

Syed, T.A., Ahmad Ashfares, Holt,
A.H., Ahmad Seyed, A., Ahmad,
S.H. & Afzal, M.
*Management of psoriasis with aloe
vera cream*
Tropical Medicine And International
Health 1996, 1(4) pp505-509

Rampton *et al.*
Ulcerative colitis
Alimentary Pharmacology And
Therapeutics 2004, Apr; 19(7):
739-747

Bland, J.
*Effect of orally consumed aloe vera
juice on gastrointestinal function in
normal humans.*
Linus Pauling Institute Of Science
And Medicine Palo Alto, C.A.
Prevention Magazine 1985

Syed, T.A. *et al.*
*Management of psoriasis with aloe
vera extract in a hydrophilic cream:
a placebo controlled double blind
study*
Tropical Medicine And
International health 1(4): 505-509
(1996)

About the author

Following a 30-year career in general practice, with a special interest in dermatology, Dr. Peter Atherton attended Oxford University as a Visiting Research Fellow at Green College. There he studied the medicinal qualities of Aloe Vera. After this period of study he wrote the definitive book on the subject *The Essential Aloe Vera.*

Dr. Atherton is Medical Advisor to Forever Living Products (U.K.) Ltd., the world's largest producer of aloe vera. Because of his expert knowledge on the subject he is invited to lecture both nationally and internationally.

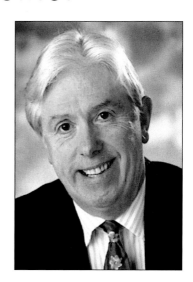

Other titles in the series

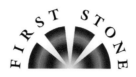

First published 2005 by First Stone Publishing
PO Box 8, Lydney, Gloucestershire, GL15 6YD

The contents of this book are for information only and are not intended as a substitute for appropriate medical attention. The author and publishers admit no liability for any consequences arising from following any advice contained within this book. If you have any concerns about your health or medication, always consult your doctor.

ISBN 1 904439 33 0

Printed and bound in China